C000021729

The Essential Keto Chaffle

Recipe Book

50 amazing recipes to

delight every day

Catherine Willis

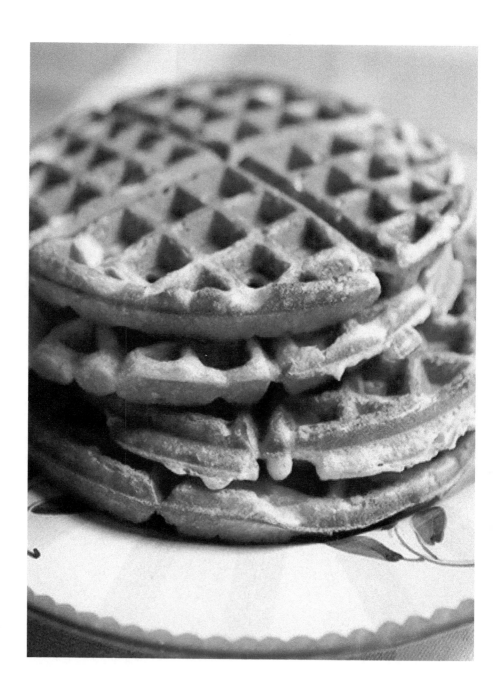

sources. Please consult a licensed professional before attempting any techniques outlined in this book.

By reading this document, the reader agrees that under no circumstances is the author responsible for any losses, direct or indirect, which are incurred as a result of the use of information contained within this document, including, but not limited to, — errors, omissions, or inaccuracies.

Table of Contents

Chocolate Chip Chaffle Keto Recipe

Prep Time: 5 mins

Cook Time: 8 mins

Serving: 1

INGREDIENTS:

1 3/4 tsp Lakanto monk fruit

golden pinch of salt

1 tbsp Lily's Chocolate Chips

1 tbsp heavy whipping cream

1/2 tsp coconut flour

1 egg

DIRECTIONS :

Switch the waffle maker on so it can heat up.

Add all ingredients in a container except the chocolate chips and stir well until mixed. Grease the waffle maker, then spill half the batter onto the waffle maker's bottom plate. Sprinkle on top with a few chocolate chips and then close.

Cook for 3-4 minutes or until the dessert of the chocolate chip chaffle is golden brown, then remove it with a fork from the waffle maker, taking care not to burn your fingers.

Repeat with the batter for the remainder.

For a few minutes, let the chaffle sit so that it starts to crisp. Serve with sugar-free whipped topping if needed

NUTRITION :

Carbohydrates: 7g Calories: 146kcal Fat: 10g Protein: 6g

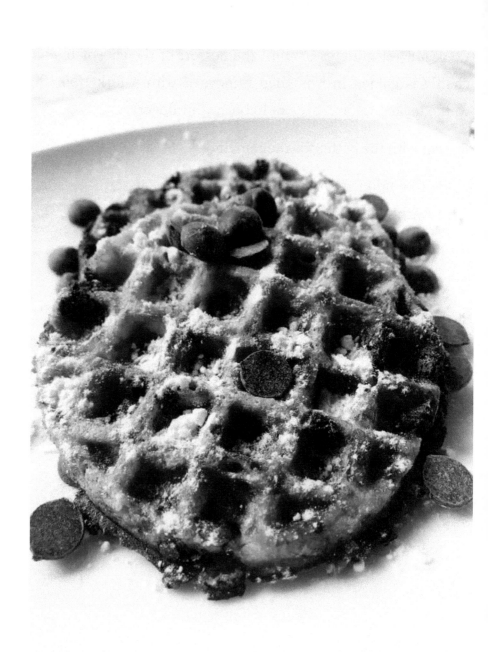

Keto Blueberry Chaffle

Prep Time: 3 minutes

Cook Time: 15 minutes

Servings : 5

INGREDIENTS:

1 cup of mozzarella cheese

2 tablespoons almond flour

1 tsp baking powder

2 eggs

1 tsp cinnamon

2 tsp of Swerve

3 tablespoon blueberries

DIRECTIONS :

Heat up your mini waffle maker.

Add the mozzarella cheese, almond flour, baking powder, eggs, cinnamon, and blueberries to the mixing bowl. Mix all of the ingredients thoroughly.

With nonstick cooking oil, spray your mini waffle maker.

A little less than 1/4 of a cup of blueberry keto waffle batter is added.

For 3-5 minutes, cover and cook the chaffle. To see if it is crispy and brown, check it at the 3 minute mark. Cover and cook for 1-2 minutes longer if it is not or it sticks to the top of the waffle machine.

Serve with a sprinkle of sugar or keto syrup for swerve confectioners.

NUTRITION :

Calories: 116kcal Carbohydrates: 3g Protein: 8g Fat: 8g

Crispy Chaffles With Egg & Asparagus

Servings:1

Cooking Time : 10 Minutes

INGREDIENTS:

1 egg

1/4 cup cheddar cheese

2 tbsps. almond flour

½ tsp. baking powder

TOPPING

1 egg

4-5 stalks asparagus

1 tsp avocado oil

DIRECTIONS :

1. Preheat the waffle maker to medium-high heat.

2. Beat egg, mozzarella cheese, almond flour, and baking powder

3. Pour chaffles mixture into the center of the waffle iron. Cover and let cook for 5 minutes or until the waffle is golden brown and set.

4. Remove chaffles from the waffle maker and serve.

5. Meanwhile, heat oil in a nonstick pan.

6. Once the pan is hot, fry asparagus for about 4-5 minutes until golden brown.

7. Poach the egg in boiling water for about 2-3 minutes.

8. Once chaffles are cooked, remove from the maker.

9. Serve chaffles with the poached egg and asparagus.

NUTRITION :

Protein: 85kcal Fat: 226kcal Carbohydrates: 16kcal

Cinnamon Roll Chaffles

Servings : 3

Prep time : 15 min.

Cook time : 25 min.

INGREDIENTS

FOR THE BATTER:

½ cup shredded mozzarella cheese

2 Tbsp golden monk fruit sweetener

2 Tbsp SunButter

1 egg

1 Tbsp coconut flour

2 tsp cinnamon

¼ tsp vanilla extract

⅛ tsp baking powder

FOR THE FROSTING:

¼ cup powdered monk fruit sweetener

1 Tbsp cream cheese

¾ Tbsp butter, melted

¼ tsp vanilla extract

1 Tbsp unsweetened coconut milk

FOR THE COATING

1 tsp cinnamon

1 tsp golden monk fruit sweetener

DIRECTIONS :

Turn on the waffle maker to heat and oil it with cooking spray.

Combine all battery components in a bowl, then set aside and leave for 3-5 minutes. In another bowl, whisk all frosting components until well-combined.

Divide batter into 3 portions and spoon 1 part into the waffle maker. Cook for 2-4 minutes, until golden brown.

Open and let the chaffle cool for 30 seconds in the waffle maker before you transfer it to a plate. Repeat with remaining batter.

While chaffles are warm, sprinkle with cinnamon and sweetener coating. When cooled a little, drizzle with icing.

NUTRITION :

Carbs – 31g Fat – 15g Protein – 9g Calories – 195

Yogurt Chaffles

Servings : 3

Prep time : 5 min. + overnight

Cook time : 10 min.

INGREDIENTS

½ cup shredded mozzarella

1 egg

2 Tbsp ground almonds

½ tsp psyllium husk

¼ tsp baking powder

1 Tbsp yogurt

DIRECTIONS :

Turn on the waffle maker to heat and oil it with cooking spray. Whisk eggs in a bowl.

Add in remaining ingredients except mozzarella and mix well. Add mozzarella and mix once again. Let it sit for 5 minutes. Add ⅓cup batter into each waffle mold.

Close and cook for 4-5 minutes.

Repeat with remaining batter.

NUTRITION :

Carbs 2g Fat 5g Protein 4gCalories 93

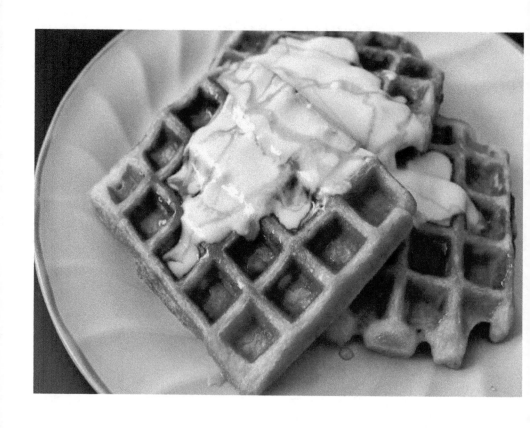

Raspberry Chaffles

Servings : 2

Prep time : 5 min.

Cook time : 5 min.

INGREDIENTS

4 Tbsp almond flour

4 large eggs

2 ⅓cup shredded mozzarella cheese

1 tsp vanilla extract

1 Tbsp erythritol sweetener

1½ tsp baking powder

½ cup raspberries

DIRECTIONS :

Turn on the waffle maker to heat and oil it with cooking spray.

Mix almond flour, sweetener, and baking powder in a bowl.

Add cheese, eggs, and vanilla extract, and mix until well-combined.

Add 1 portion of batter to the waffle maker and spread it evenly. Close and cook for 3-4 minutes, or until golden.

Repeat until remaining batter is used. Serve with raspberries.

NUTRITION :

Carbs 4g Fat 1g Protein 6g Calories 73

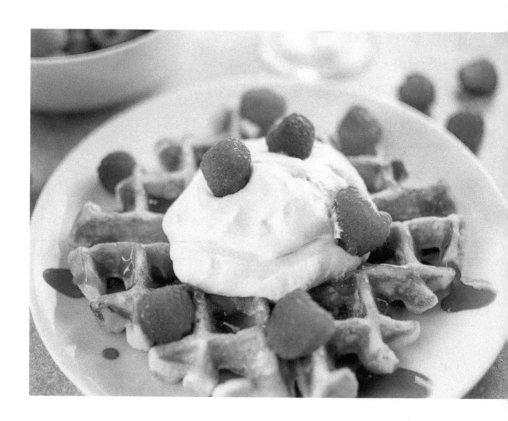

Coconut Chaffles

Servings : 2

Cooking Time : 5 Minutes

INGREDIENTS:

1 egg

1 oz. cream cheese,

1 oz. cheddar cheese

2 tbsps. coconut flour

1 tsp. stevia

1 tbsp. coconut oil, melted

1/2 tsp. coconut extract

2 eggs, soft boil for serving

DIRECTIONS :

1. Heat your minutesi Dash waffle maker and grease with cooking spray.

2. Mix together all chaffles ingredients in a bowl.

3. Pour chaffle batter in a preheated waffle maker.

4. Cover.

5. Cook chaffles for about 2-3 minutes until golden brown.

6. Serve with boiled egg and enjoy!

NUTRITION :

Protein: 32kcal Fat: 117kcal Carbohydrates: 4kcal

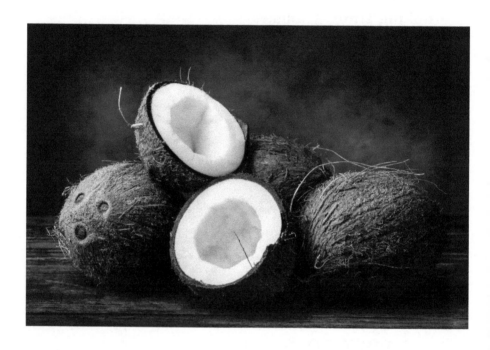

Garlic And Parsley Chaffles

Servings :1

Cooking Time : 5 Minutes

INGREDIENTS:

1 large egg

1/4 cup cheese mozzarella

1 tsp. coconut flour

¼ tsp. baking powder

½ tsp. garlic powder

1 tbsp. minutesced parsley

For Serving

1 Poach egg

4 oz. smoked salmon

DIRECTIONS :

1. Switch on yourDash minutes waffle maker and let it preheat.

2. Grease waffle maker with cooking spray.

3. Mix together egg, mozzarella, coconut flour, baking powder, and garlic powder, parsley to a mixing bowl until combined well.

4. Pour batter in circle waffle maker.

5. Cover.

6. Cook until the chaffles are done, about 2-3 minutes.

7. Serve with smoked salmon and poached egg.

NUTRITION :

Protein: 140 kcal Fat: 160kcal Carbohydrates: 14kcal

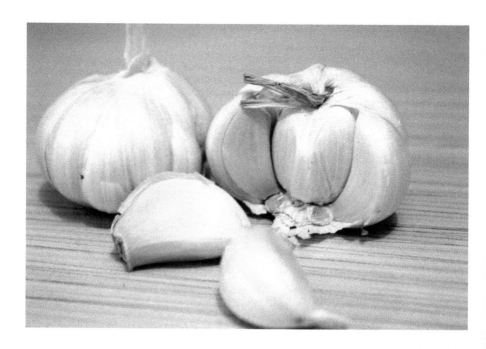

Scrambled Eggs On A Spring Onion Chaffle

Servings :4

Cooking Time : 7-9 Minutes

INGREDIENTS:

Batter

4 eggs

2 cups grated mozzarella cheese

Salt and pepper

½ teaspoon dried garlic powder

2 tablespoons almond flour

2 spring onions, finely chopped

2 tablespoons coconut flour

2 tablespoons butter for brushing the waffle maker

6-8 eggs

Salt and pepper

1 teaspoon Italian spice mix

1 tablespoon olive oil

1 tablespoon freshly chopped parsley

DIRECTIONS :

1. Preheat the waffle maker.

2. Break the eggs and add the grated cheese in a bowl.

3. Mix until just combined, then add the chopped spring onions and season with salt and pepper and dried garlic powder.

4. Stir in the almond flour and mix thoroughly.

5. Rub butter on the heated waffle maker and add a few tablespoons of the batter.

6.Cover and cook for about 7-8 minutes.

7. While the chaffles are cooking, prepare the scrambled eggs by whisking the eggs in a bowl until frothy. To taste, season with salt and black pepper and add the Italian spice mix. Whisk to blend in the spices.

8. Warm the oil in a non-stick pan over medium heat.

9. Pour the eggs in the pan and cook until eggs are set to your liking.

10. Serve each chaffle and top with some scrambled eggs. Top with freshly chopped parsley.

NUTRITION :

Calories 194, fat 14.7g, carbs 5g, Protein 1g

Strawberry Shortcake Chaffles

Servings : 1

Prep time : 20 min.

Cook time : 25 min.

INGREDIENTS

FOR THE BATTER:

1 egg

¼ cup mozzarella cheese

1 Tbsp cream cheese

¼ tsp baking powder

2 strawberries, sliced

1 tsp strawberry extract

FOR THE GLAZE:

1 Tbsp cream cheese

¼ tsp strawberry extract

1 Tbsp monk fruit confectioners blend

FOR THE WHIPPED CREAM:

1 cup heavy whipping cream

1 tsp vanilla

1 Tbsp monk fruit

DIRECTIONS :

Turn on the waffle maker to heat and oil it with cooking spray. Beat egg in a small bowl.

Add remaining batter components. Divide the mixture in half.

Cook one half of the batter in a waffle maker for 4 minutes, or until golden brown. Repeat with remaining batter

Mix all glaze ingredients and spread over each warm chaffle. Mix all whipped cream ingredients and whip until it starts to form peaks. Top each waffle with whipped cream and strawberries.

NUTRITION :

Carbs 5g Fat 14gProtein 12gCalories 218

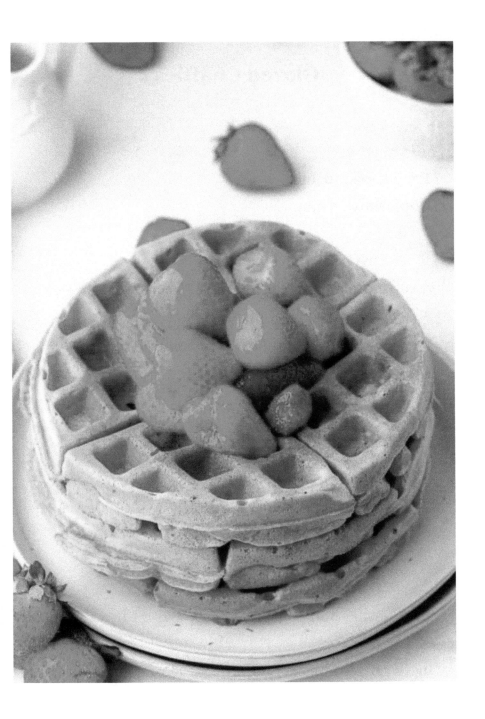

Glazed Chaffles

Servings : 2

Prep time : 10 min.

Cook time : 5 min.

INGREDIENTS :

½ cup mozzarella shredded cheese ⅛ cup cream cheese

2 Tbsp unflavored whey protein isolate

2 Tbsp swerve confectioners sugar substitute ½ tsp baking powder

½ tsp vanilla extract

1 egg

FOR THE GLAZE TOPPING:

2 Tbsp heavy whipping cream

3-4 Tbsp swerve confectioners sugar substitute ½ tsp vanilla extract

DIRECTIONS :

Turn on the waffle maker to heat and oil it with cooking spray.

In a microwave-safe bowl, mix mozzarella and cream cheese.

Heat at half minute intervals until melted and fully combined.

Add protein, 2 Tbsp sweetener, baking powder to cheese. Knead with hands until well incorporated. Place dough into a mixing bowl and beat in egg and vanilla until a smooth batter forms.

Put ⅓of the batter into the waffle maker, and cook for 3-5 minutes, until golden brown. Repeat until all 3 chaffles are made.

Beat glaze ingredients in a bowl and pour over chaffles before serving.

NUTRITION :

Carbs 4g Fat 6gProtein 4gCalories 130

Cream Mini-Chaffles

Servings : 2

Prep time : 5 min.

Cook time : 10 min.

INGREDIENTS :

2 tsp coconut flour

4 tsp swerve/monk fruit

¼ tsp baking powder

1 egg

1 oz cream cheese

½ tsp vanilla extract

DIRECTIONS :

Turn on the waffle maker to heat and oil it with cooking spray.

Mix swerve/monk fruit, coconut flour, and baking powder in a small mixing bowl. Add cream cheese, egg, vanilla extract, and whisk until well-combined.

Add batter into the waffle maker and cook for 3-4 minutes, until golden brown. Serve with your favorite toppings.

NUTRITION :

Carbs 4gFat 6gProtein 2gCalories 73

Lemon Curd Chaffles

Servings : 1

prep time : 45 min.

Cook time : 5 min.

INGREDIENTS :

3 large eggs

4 oz cream cheese, softened

1 Tbsp low carb sweetener

1 tsp vanilla extract

¾ cup mozzarella cheese, shredded

3 Tbsp coconut flour

1 tsp baking powder

⅓ tsp salt

FOR THE LEMON CURD:

½-1 cup water

5 egg yolks

½ cup lemon juice

½ cup powdered sweetener

2 Tbsp fresh lemon zest

1 tsp vanilla extract Pinch of salt

8 Tbsp cold butter, cubed

DIRECTIONS :

Pour water into a saucepan and heat over medium until it reaches a soft boil. Start with ½ cup and add more if needed.

Whisk yolks, lemon juice, lemon zest, powdered sweetener, vanilla, and salt in a medium heat-proof bowl. Leave to set for 5-6 minutes.

Place bowl onto saucepan and heat. The bowl shouldn't be touching water. Whisk mixture for 8-10 minutes, or until it begins to thicken.

Add butter cubes and whisk for 5-7 minutes, until it thickens. When it lightly coats the back of a spoon, remove from heat. Refrigerate until cool, allowing it to continue thickening.

Turn on the waffle maker to heat and oil it with cooking spray.

Add baking powder, coconut flour, and salt in a small bowl. Mix well and set aside.

Add eggs, cream cheese, sweetener, and vanilla in a separate bowl. Using a hand beater, beat until frothy.

Add mozzarella to the egg mixture and beat again.

Add dry **INGREDIENTS** and mix until well-combined.

Add batter to the waffle maker and cook for 3-4 minutes.

Transfer to a plate and top with lemon curd before serving

NUTRITION :

Carbs 6g Fat 24gProtein 15gCalories 302

Egg On A Cheddar Cheese Chaffle

Servings : 4

Cooking Time : 7-9 Minutes

INGREDIENTS :

Batter

4 eggs

2 cups shredded white cheddar cheese Salt and pepper to taste

Other

2 tablespoons butter for brushing the waffle maker

4 large eggs

2 tablespoons olive oil

DIRECTIONS :

1. Preheat the waffle maker.

2. Break And whisk the eggs into a bowl with a fork.

3. Stir in the grated cheddar cheese and season with salt and pepper.

4. Rub butter on the heated waffle maker and add a few tablespoons of the batter.

5. Cover and cook for about 7-8 minutes depending on your waffle maker.

6. While chaffles are cooking, cook the eggs.

7. Heat the oil for 2-3 minutes over medium-low heat in a large non-stick pan with a lid.

8. Break an egg and gently add it to the pan. Repeat the same way for the other 3 eggs.

9. Cover and let cook for 2 to 2 ½ minutes for set eggs but with runny yolks.

10. Remove from heat.

11. To serve, place a chaffle on each plate and top with an egg. To taste season with salt and black pepper.

NUTRITION :

Calories 4 fat 34g, carbs 2g, sugar 0.6g,Protein 26g

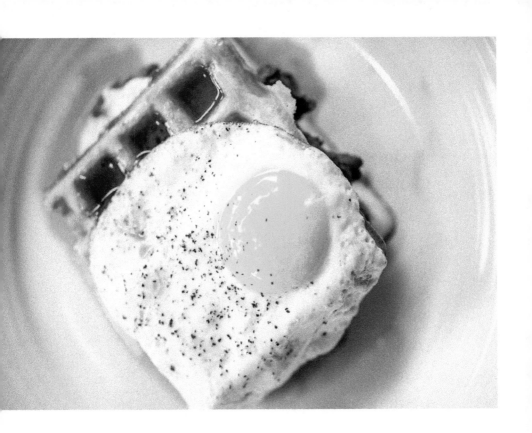

Avocado Chaffle Toast

Servings : 3

Cooking Time : 10 Minutes

INGREDIENTS :

4 tbsps. avocado mash

1/2 tsp lemon juice

1/8 tsp salt

1/8 tsp black pepper

2 eggs

1/2 cup shredded cheese

For serving

3 eggs

½ avocado thinly sliced

1 tomato, sliced

DIRECTIONS :

1. Mash avocado mash with lemon juice, salt, and black pepper in a mixing bowl, until well combined.

2. In a small bowl beat egg and pour eggs in avocado mixture and mix well.

3. Switch on Waffle Maker to pre-heat.

4. Pour 1/8 of shredded cheese in a waffle maker and then pour ½ of egg and avocado mixture and then 1/8 shredded cheese.

5. Cover and cook chaffles for about 3 - 4 minutes.

6. Repeat with the remaining mixture.

7. Meanwhile,fry eggs in a pan for about 1-2 minutes.

8. For serving, arrange fried egg on chaffle toast with avocado slice and tomatoes.

9. Sprinkle salt and pepper on top and enjoy!

NUTRITION :

Protein: 66kcal Fat: 169kcal Carbohydrates: 15kcal

Cajun & Feeta Chaffles

Servings : 1

Cooking Time : 10 Minutes

INGREDIENTS :

1 egg white

1/4 cup shredded mozzarella cheese

2 tbsps. almond flour

1 tsp Cajun Seasoning

FOR SERVING

1 egg

4 oz. feta cheese

1 tomato, sliced

DIRECTIONS :

1. Whisk together egg, cheese, and seasoning in a bowl.

2. Switch on and grease waffle maker with cooking spray.

3. Pour batter in a preheated waffle maker.

4. Cook chaffles for about 2-3 minutes until the chaffle is cooked through.

5. Meanwhile, fry the egg in a non-stick pan for about 1-2 minutes.

6. For serving, set fried egg on chaffles with feta cheese and tomato slices.

NUTRITION :

Protein: 119kcal Fat 2kcal Carbohydrates: 31kcal

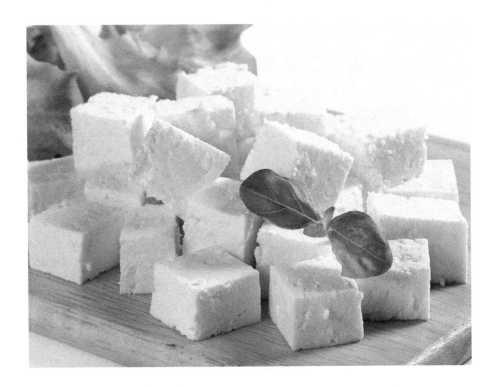

Crispy Waffles With Sausage

Servings :2

Cooking Time : 10 Minutes

INGREDIENTS :

1/2 cup cheddar cheese

1/2 tsp. baking powder

1/4 cup egg whites

2 tsp. pumpkin spice

1 egg, whole

2 chicken sausage

2 slice bacon

salt and pepper to taste

1 tsp. avocado oil

DIRECTIONS :

1. Mix together all **INGREDIENTS** in a bowl.

2. Allow batter to sit while waffle iron warms.

3. Spray waffle iron with nonstick spray.

4. Add the batter and cook in the waffle maker.

5. Meanwhile, heat oil in a pan and fry the egg.

6. In the same pan, fry bacon slices and sausage on medium heat for about 2-3 minutes until cooked.

7. Once chaffles are cooked thoroughly, remove them from the maker.

8. Serve with fried egg, bacon slice, sausages and enjoy!

NUTRITION :

Calories 208 Fat 13.5g Carbohydrate 0.7g Protein 8.2g Sugars 0.6g

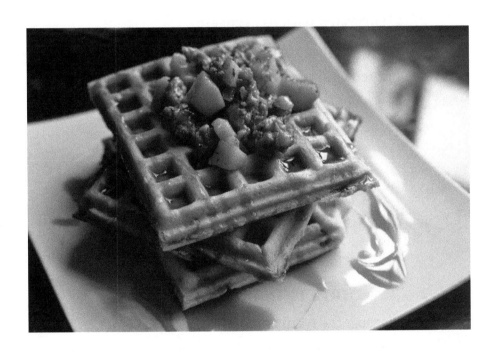

Chili Chaffle

Servings :4

Cooking Time :7-9 Minutes

INGREDIENTS :

Batter

4 eggs

½ cup grated parmesan cheese

1½ cups grated yellow cheddar cheese

1 hot red chili pepper

Salt and pepper to taste

½ teaspoon dried garlic powder

1 teaspoon dried basil

2 tablespoons almond flour

Other

2 tablespoons olive oil for brushing the waffle maker

DIRECTIONS :

1. Preheat the waffle maker.

2. Break the eggs into a bowl and add the grated parmesan and cheddar cheese.

3. Mix until just combined and add the chopped chili pepper. Season with salt and pepper, dried garlic powder and dried basil. Stir in the almond flour.

4. Mix until everything is combined.

5. Brush the heated waffle maker with olive oil and add a few tablespoons of the batter.

6. Cover and cook for about 7-8 minutes depending on your waffle maker.

NUTRITION :

Calories 36 fat 30.4g, carbs 3.1g

Simple Savory Chaffle

Servings :4

Cooking Time : 7-9 Minutes

INGREDIENTS :

Batter

4 eggs

1 cup grated mozzarella cheese

1 cup grated provolone cheese ½ cup almond flour

2 tablespoons coconut flour

2½ teaspoons baking powder

Salt and pepper to taste

2 tablespoons butter

DIRECTIONS :

1. Preheat the waffle maker.

2. Add the grated mozzarella and provolone cheese to a bowl and mix.

3. Add the almond and coconut flour and baking powder and season with salt and pepper.

4. Mix with a wire whisk and crack in the eggs.

5. Stir everything together until the batter forms.

6. Rub butter on the heated waffle maker and add a few tablespoons of the batter.

7. Cover and cook for about 8 minutes.

8. Serve and enjoy.

NUTRITION :

Calories 352, fat 27.2g, carbs 8.3g, Protein 15g

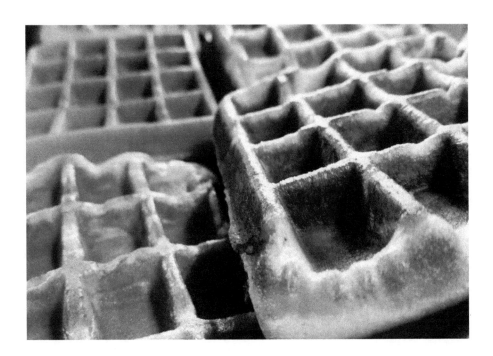

Pizza Chaffle

Servings :4

Cooking Time :7-9 Minutes

INGREDIENTS :

Batter

4 eggs

1½ cups grated mozzarella cheese

½ cup grated parmesan cheese

2 tablespoons tomato sauce ¼ cup almond flour

1½ teaspoons baking powder

Salt and pepper to taste

1 teaspoon dried oregano

¼ cup sliced salami

Other

2 tablespoons olive oil for brushing the waffle maker ¼ cup tomato sauce for serving

DIRECTIONS :

1. Preheat the waffle maker.

2. Add the grated mozzarella and grated parmesan to a bowl and mix.

3. Add the almond flour and baking powder and season with salt and pepper and dried oregano.

4. Mix and smash the eggs with a wooden spoon or wire whisk.

5. Stir everything together until the batter forms.

6. Stir in the chopped salami.

7. Brush the heated waffle maker with olive oil and add a few tablespoons of the batter.

8. Cover and cook for about 7-minutes depending on your waffle maker.

9. Serve with extra tomato sauce on top and enjoy.

NUTRITION :

Calories 319, fat 25.2g, carbs 5.9g, Protein 19.3g

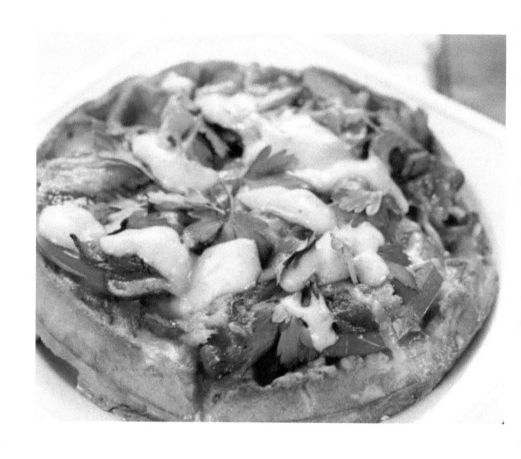

Bacon Chaffle

Servings :4

Cooking Time :7-9 Minutes

INGREDIENTS :

Batter

4 eggs

2 cups shredded mozzarella

2 ounces finely chopped bacon Salt and pepper to taste

1 teaspoon dried oregano

2 tablespoons olive oil for brushing the waffle maker

DIRECTIONS :

1. Preheat the waffle maker.

2. Break the eggs into a bowl and add the grated mozzarella cheese.

3. Mix until just combined and stir in the chopped bacon.

4. Season with salt and pepper and dried oregano.

5. Rub olive oil on the heated waffle maker and add a few tablespoons of the batter.

6. Cover and cook for about 7-8 minutes depending on your waffle maker.

NUTRITION :

Calories 241, fat 19.8g, carbs 1.3g,Protein 14.8g

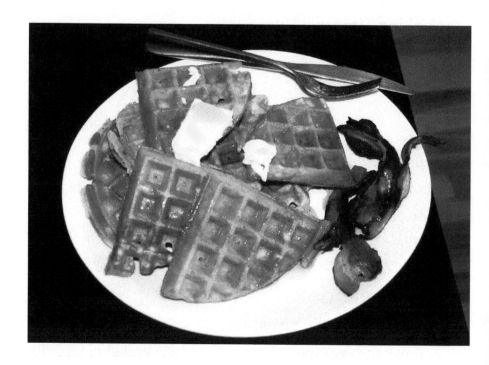

Chaffles Breakfast Bowl

Servings :2

Cooking Time : 5 Minutes

INGREDIENTS :

1/2 cup cheddar cheese shredded

pinch of Italian seasoning

1 tbsp. pizza sauce

1 egg

TOPPING

1/2 avocado sliced

2 eggs boiled

1 tomato, halves

4 oz. fresh spinach leaves

DIRECTIONS :

1. Preheat your waffle maker and grease with cooking spray.

2. Crack an egg in a small bowl and beat with Italian seasoning and pizza sauce.

3. Add shredded cheese to the egg and spices mixture.

4. Pour 1 tbsp. shredded cheese in a waffle maker and cook for 30 sec.

5. Pour Waffles batter in the waffle maker and cover.

6. Cook chaffles for about 4 minutes until crispy and brown.

7. Carefully remove chaffles from the maker.

8. Serve on the bed of spinach with boiled egg, avocado slice, and tomatoes.

9. Enjoy!

NUTRITION :

Protein: 77kcal Fat: 222kcal Carbohydrates: 39kcal

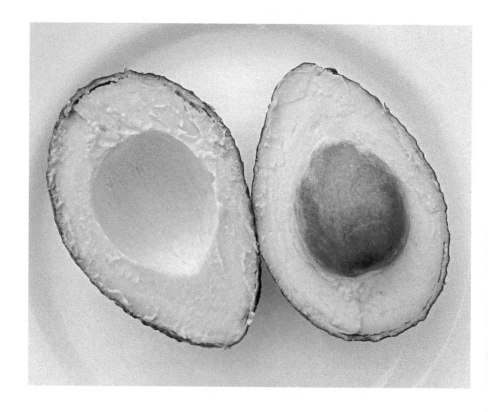

Morning Chaffles With Berries

Servings : 4

Cooking Time : 5 Minutes

INGREDIENTS :

1 cup egg whites

1 cup cheddar cheese, shredded ¼ cup almond flour

¼ cup heavy cream

TOPPING

4 oz. raspberries

4 oz. strawberries.

1 oz. keto chocolate flakes

1 oz. feta cheese.

DIRECTIONS :

1. Preheat your square waffle maker and grease with cooking spray.

2. Crack egg white with flour in a small bowl.

3. Add shredded cheese to the egg whites and flour mixture and mix well.

4. Add cream and cheese to the egg mixture.

5. Pour Chaffles batter in a waffle maker and cover.

6. Cook chaffles for about 4 minutes until crispy and brown.

7. Carefully remove chaffles from the maker.

8. Serve with berries, cheese, and chocolate on top.

9. Enjoy!

NUTRITION :

Protein: 68kcal Fat: 163kcal Carbohydrates: 12kcal

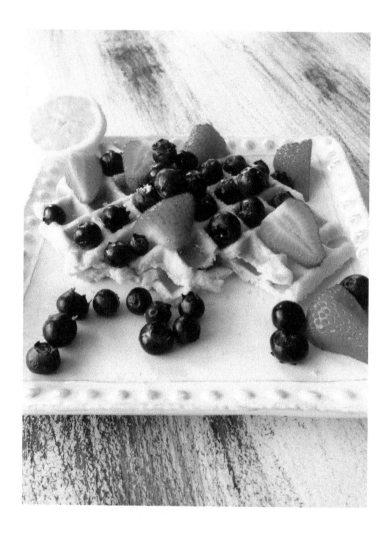

Chocolate Vanilla Chaffles

Servings : 2

Prep time: 5 min.

Cook time: 5 min.

INGREDIENTS :

½ cup shredded mozzarella cheese

1 egg

1 Tbsp granulated sweetener

1 tsp vanilla extract

1 Tbsp sugar-free chocolate chips

2 Tbsp almond meal/flour

DIRECTIONS :

Turn on the waffle maker to heat and oil it with cooking spray. Mix all components in a bowl until combined.

Introduce half of the batter into the waffle maker.

Cook for 2-4 minutes, then remove and repeat with remaining batter. Top with more chips and favorite toppings.

NUTRITION :

Carbs 23g Fat 3g Protein 4gCalories 134

Keto Chaffle Breakfast Sandwich

Prep Time : 3 minutes
Cook Time : 6 minutes
Servings : 1

INGREDIENTS :

1 tablespoon almond flour

1/2 cup Monterey Jack Cheese

2 tablespoons butter

1 egg

DIRECTIONS :

Combine egg, almond flour, and Monterey Jack Cheese in a small cup.

Through your mini waffle maker, add half the batter and cook for 3-4 minutes. To make a second chaffle, then cook the rest of the batter.

In a small pan, liquified 2 tablespoons of butter. Attach the chaffles and cook them for 2 minutes on each side.

Take out of the pan and let sit for 2 minutes.

NUTRITION :

Carbohydrates: 2g Protein: 21g Fat: 47g Calories: 514kca l

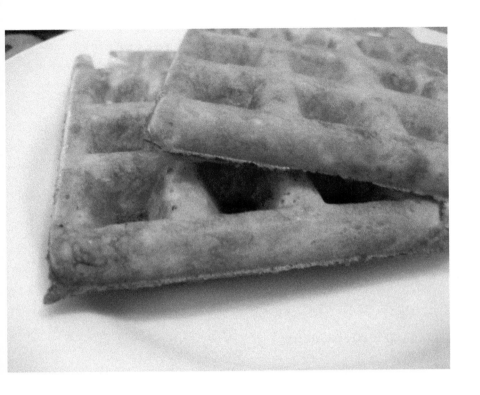

Keto Chaffle Taco Shells

Prep Time : 5 minutes

Cook Time : 20 minutes

Servings : 5

INGREDIENTS :

1 tablespoon almond flour

1 cup taco blend cheese

2 eggs

1/4 tsp taco seasoning

DIRECTIONS :

Combine the almond flour, taco cheese mix, eggs, and taco seasoning in a dish. Using a fork, I find it best to combine anything.

Introduce 1.5 tablespoons of taco chaffle batter at a time to the waffle maker; cook 4 minutes of chaffle batter in the waffle maker.

Remove the waffle maker's taco chaffle shell and drape it over the side of a tub.

Keep making taco chaffle shells until you're out of the batter. Then fill the taco shells with taco meat, and enjoy your favorite toppings!

NUTRITION :

Calories: 113kcal Protein: 8g Carbohydrates: 1g Fat: 9g

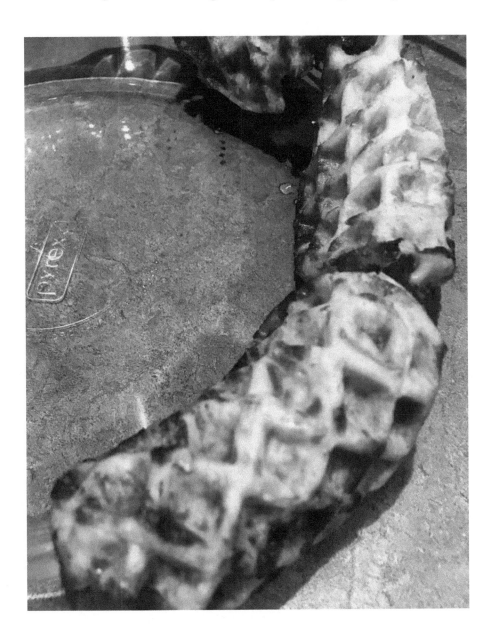

Peanut Butter Chaffle

Prep Time : 3 minutes
Cook Time : 8 minutes
Servings : 2

INGREDIENTS :

1 egg

1/2 cup mozzarella cheese shredded

3 tablespoons swerve granulated

2 tbsp peanut butter

DIRECTIONS :

Heat up the waffle maker.

Combine the peanut butter, bacon, pellet swerve and mozzarella cheese in a dish.

Into the waffle maker, add half the chaffle batter and cook for 4 minutes.

When cooked, carefully remove it and put it on a plate to cool. When you remove it, the chaffle will be a little flimsy, but when it cools, it will stiffen up.

First, cook your second chaffle and after you cook it, let it sit for 2 minutes.

NUTRITION :

Carbohydrates: 4g Protein: 13g Fat: 16g Calories: 210kcal

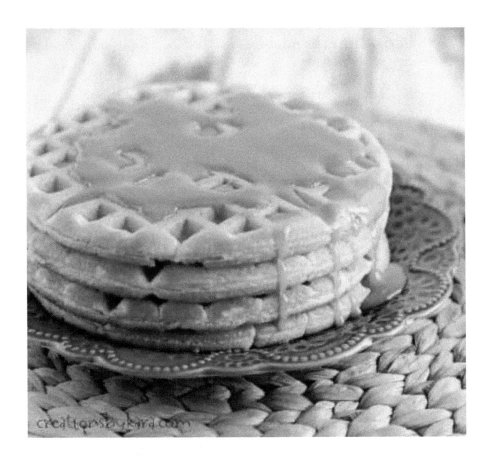

Pumpkin Chocolate Chip Waffles

Prep Time : 4 minutes

Cook Time: 12 minutes

Servings : 3

INGREDIENTS :

1/2 cup shredded mozzarella cheese

4 teaspoons pumpkin puree

1 egg

2 tablespoons granulated Swerve 1/4 tsp pumpkin pie spice

4 teaspoons sugar-free chocolate chips

1 tablespoon almond flour

DIRECTIONS :

Plug in your waffle maker.

Mix the pumpkin puree and egg in a bowl. Make sure you mix it well, so all the pumpkin is mixed with the egg.

Next, add in the mozzarella cheese, almond flour, swerve and add pumpkin spice and mix well. Then add in your sugar-free chocolate chips

Add half of the Chaffle mix keto pumpkin pie to the Dish Mini waffle maker at a time. In a waffle maker, cook the chaffle batter for 4 minutes.

Do not open up until 4 minutes have passed.

Cook the second one when the first one is fully finished.

Enjoy sweetener or whipped cream on top with a few swerve confectioners.

NUTRITION :

Calories: 93kcal Carbohydrates: 2g Protein: 7g Fat: 7g

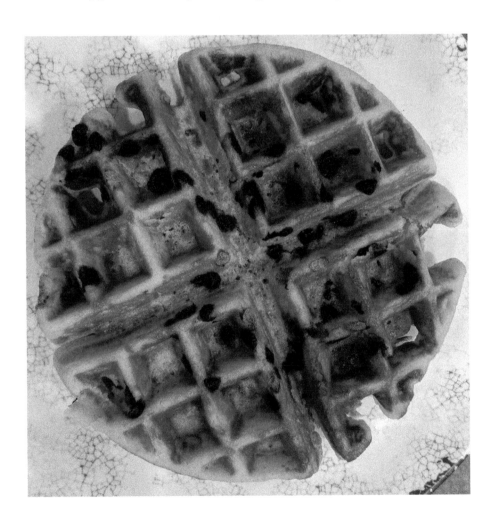

Broccoli & Cheese Chaffle

Prep Time : 2 minutes

Cook Time : 8 minutes

Servings : 2

INGREDIENTS :

1/2 cup cheddar cheese

1/4 cup fresh chopped broccoli

1 egg

1/4 teaspoon garlic powder

1 tablespoon almond flour

DIRECTIONS :

Mix the almond flour, cheddar cheese, egg, and garlic powder together in a dish.

To the Dish Mini waffle maker, add half of the broccoli and cheese waffle batter at a time. In a waffle maker, cook the chaffle batter for 4 minutes.

Let each chaffle settle on a plate for 1-2 minutes to firm up. Enjoy yourself or roll yourself in sour cream or ranch dressing.

NUTRITION :

Carbohydrates: 2g Protein: 11g Fat: 13g Calories: 170kcal

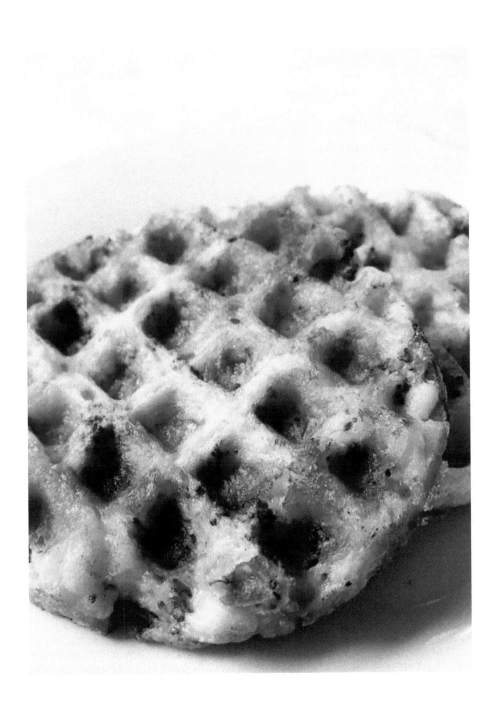

French Dip Keto Waffle Sandwich

Prep Time : 5 mins

Cook Time : 12 mins

Servings : 2

INGREDIENTS :

1 egg white

1/4 cup sharp cheddar cheese, shredded

3/4 tsp water

1/4 tsp baking powder

1/4 cup mozzarella cheese, shredded (packed)

Pinch of salt

1 tsp coconut flour

DIRECTIONS :

Preheat the oven to 425°C. Once it is warmed, plug the Dash Mini Waffle Maker into the wall and lightly grease it.

In a bowl, combine all the ingredients and mix to combine.

Spoon out 1/2 of the batter and cover on the waffle maker. Set a timer for 4 minutes and until the cooking time is full, do not raise the lid.

From the waffle iron, remove the chaffle and set aside. For the remainder of the chaffle batter, repeat the same steps above.

Use parchment paper to cover a cookie sheet and put chaffles a few inches apart.

From the following recipe, add 1/4 to 1/3 cup of slow cooker keto roast beef.

On top of that, add a slice of deli cheese or shredded cheese. To allow the cheese to melt, place it on the top rack of the oven for 5 minutes.

Enjoy with a small bowl of beef broth open-faced for dipping.

NUTRITION :

Carbohydrates: 2g Protein: 9g Fat: 8g Calories: 118kcal

Fudgy Chocolate Chaffles

Prep Time: 5 mins
Cook Time : 8 mins
Servings : 2

INGREDIENTS :

1 egg

2 tbsp mozzarella cheese, shredded

2 tbsp cocoa

2 tbsp Lakanto monk fruit powdered

1 tsp coconut flour

1 tsp heavy whipping cream

1/4 tsp baking powder

1/4 tsp vanilla extract

pinch of salt

DIRECTIONS :

Switch on the chaffle or waffle maker. Lightly grease or use cooking spray.

Combine every ingredient in a small bowl

Cover with 1/2 of the batter for the dash mini waffle maker. Close the maker of mini waffles and cook for

With 4 minutes. Cautiously remove the chaff from the waffle maker. Repeat the above steps.

Serve with sugar-free strawberry ice cream or whipped topping without sugar.

NUTRITION :

Carbohydrates: 5g Protein: 7g Fat: 7gCalories: 109kcal

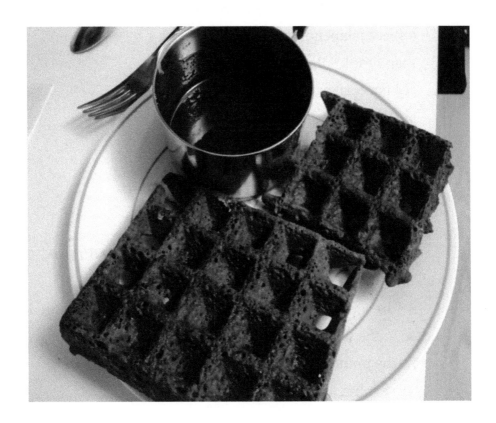

Keto Cornbread Chaffle

INGREDIENTS :

1 egg

1/2 cup cheddar cheese shredded (or mozzarella)

5 slices jalapeno - pickled or fresh

1 tsp Frank's Red hot sauce

1/4 tsp corn extract

pinch salt

DIRECTIONS :

Preheat the mini waffles maker

Whip the egg in a small bowl.

The rest of the ingredients are introduced and mixed until well integrated.

Before adding the mixture, add a teaspoon of shredded cheese to the waffle maker for 30 seconds.

To the preheated waffle maker, add half the mixture.

Serve it hot and enjoy it!

NUTRITION :

Carbohydrates: 7g Protein: 10g Fat: 7gCalories: 129kcal

Keto Chaffle Stuffing Recipe

Preparation time: 5 minutes

Cooking time: 10 minutes

Servings : 4

INGREDIENTS :

1/4 tsp garlic powder

1/2 tsp dried poultry seasoning

1/4 tsp salt

1/4 tsp pepper

2 eggs

1/2 tsp onion powder

1/2 cup cheese mozzarella, cheddar or both

STUFFING INGREDIENTS :

1 small onion diced

2 celery stalks

4 oz mushrooms diced

4 tbsp butter for sauteing

3 eggs

DIRECTIONS :

Make your chaffles first.

Preheat the iron with the mini waffle.

Preheat the furnace to 350F

Combine the chaffle components in a medium-size bowl.

In a mini waffle maker, pour 1/4 of the mixture and cook each chaffle for about 4 minutes each.

Set them aside once they are all cooked.

Saute the onion, celery, and mushrooms in a small frying pan until they are soft.

Tear the chaffles into small pieces in a separate bowl, stir in the sauteed veggies, and add 3 eggs. Mix until they are fully combined with the ingredients.

In a small casserole dish, add the stuffing mixture and bake it at 350 degrees for about 30 to 40 minutes.

Carrot Cake Chaffle

Servings : 10

Cooking Time : 18 Minutes

INGREDIENTS :

1 tbsp toasted pecans (chopped)

2 tbsp granulated swerve

1 tsp pumpkin spice

1 tsp baking powder

½ shredded carrots

2 tbsp butter (melted)

1 tsp cinnamon

1 tsp vanilla extract (optional)

2 tbsp heavy whipping cream ¾ cup almond flour

1 egg (beaten)

Butter cream cheese frosting:

½ cup cream cheese (softened)

¼ cup butter (softened)

½ tsp vanilla extract

¼ cup granulated swerve

DIRECTIONS :

1. Plug the chaffle maker to preheat it and spray it with a non-stick cooking spray.

2. In a bowl, combine the almond flour, cinnamon, carrot, pumpkin spice and swerve.

3. In a separate bowl, beat together the eggs, butter, heavy whipping cream and vanilla extract.

4. Pour the flour mixture into the egg mixture and mix until you form a smooth batter.

5. Fold in the chopped pecans.

6. Pour in an appropriate amount of the batter into your waffle maker and spread out the batter to the edges to cover all the holes on the waffle maker.

7. Cover and cook for about 3 minutes.

8. After the cooking cycle, remove the chaff from the waffle maker.

9. Repeat step 6 to 8 until you have cooked all the batter into waffles.

10. For the frosting, combine the cream cheese and cutter into a mixer and mix until well combined.

11. Add the swerve and vanilla extract and slowly until the sweetener is well incorporated. Mix on high until the frosting is fluffy.

12. Place one chaffle on a flat surface and spread some cream frosting over it. Layer another chaffle over the first one and spread some cream over it too.

13. Repeat step 12 until you have assembled all the chaffles into a cake.

14. Cut and serve.

NUTRITION :

Calories 208 Fat 13.5g Carbohydrate 0.7g Protein 8.2g
Sugars 0.6g

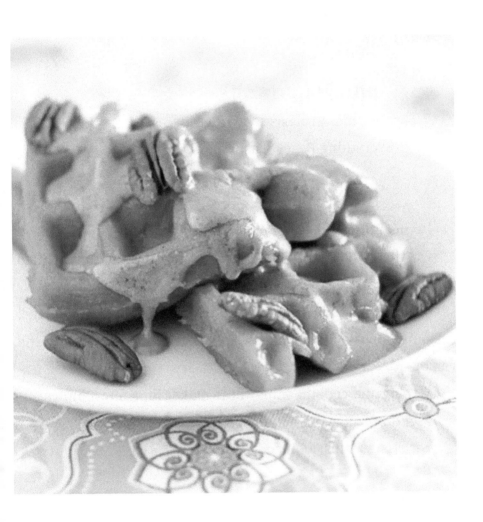

Crispy Bagel Chaffle Chips

Preparation time: 5 minutes
Cooking time: 10 minutes
Servings : 1

INGREDIENTS :

3 Tbsp Parmesan cheese shredded
1 tsp Everything Bagel Seasoning

DIRECTIONS :

Preheat the mini waffle machine

On the griddle, place the Parmesan cheese and allow it to bubble. Approximately 3 minutes.

Sprinkle with approximately 1 teaspoon of Everything Bagel Seasoning on the melted cheese. When it cooks, leave the waffle iron open!

Unplug and cool the mini waffle maker for a few minutes.

Peel the warm with a mini spatula.

For crispy chips, let it cool completely!

NUTRITION :

Total Fat 5.6g Total Carbohydrate 1.2g Protein 6.2g

Chaffle Churros

Servings : 2
Prep time : 10 min.
Cook time : 5 min.

INGREDIENTS :

1 egg

1 Tbsp almond flour

½ tsp vanilla extract

1 tsp cinnamon, divided

¼ tsp baking powder

½ cup shredded mozzarella

1 Tbsp swerve confectioners sugar substitute

1 Tbsp swerve brown sugar substitute

1 Tbsp butter, melted

DIRECTIONS :

Turn on the waffle maker to heat and oil it with cooking spray.

Mix egg, flour, vanilla extract, ½ tsp cinnamon, baking powder, mozzarella, and sugar substitute in a bowl.

Put a portion of the mixture into the waffle maker and cook for 3-5 minutes, or until desired doneness. Remove and place the second half of the batter into the maker.

Cut chaffles into strips.

Place strips in a bowl and cover with melted butter.

Mix brown sugar substitute and the remaining cinnamon in a bowl. Pour sugar mixture over the strips and toss to coat them well.

NUTRITION :

Carbs 5gFat 6gProtein 5g Calories 7 6

Cinnamon Pecan Waffles

Servings : 1

Prep time : 20 min. + 12 h.

Cook time: 40 min.

INGREDIENTS :

1 Tbsp butter

1 egg

½ tsp vanilla

2 Tbsp almond flour

1 Tbsp coconut flour

⅛ tsp baking powder

1 Tbsp monk fruit

    FOR THE CRUMBLE:

½ tsp cinnamon

1 Tbsp melted butter

1 tsp monk fruit

1 Tbsp chopped pecans

DIRECTIONS :

Turn on the waffle maker to heat and oil it with cooking spray.

In a cup, melt the butter and then add the egg and vanilla.

Mix in remaining chaffle ingredients.

Combine crumble ingredients in a separate bowl.

Introduce half of the chaffle mix into the waffle maker. Top with half of the crumble mixture. Cook for 5 minutes, or until done.

Repeat with the other half of the batter.

NUTRITION :

Carbs 8gFat 35gProtein 10gCalories 391

Oreo Keto Chaffles

Servings : 2

Prep time : 5 min.

Cook time : 5 min.

INGREDIENTS :

1 egg

1½ Tbsp unsweetened cocoa

2 Tbsp lakanto monk fruit, or choice of sweetener

1 Tbsp heavy cream

1 tsp coconut flour

½ tsp baking powder

½ tsp vanilla

FOR THE CHEESE CREAM:

1 Tbsp lakanto powdered sweetener

2 Tbsp softened cream cheese ¼ tsp vanilla

DIRECTIONS :

Turn on the waffle maker to heat and oil it with cooking spray. Combine all chaffle ingredients in a small bowl.

Pour one half of the chaffle mixture into the waffle maker. Cook for 3-5 minutes.

Remove and repeat with the second half of the mixture. Let chaffles sit for 2-3 to crisp up.

Combine all cream ingredients and spread on chaffle when they have cooled to room temperature.

NUTRITION :

Carbs 3g Fat 4gProtein 7gCalories 66

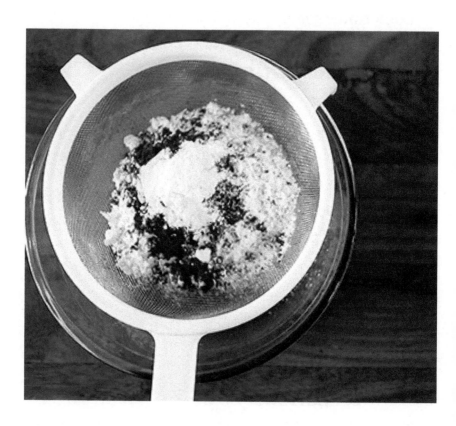

Chicken Bites With Chaffles

Servings : 2

Cooking Time : 10 minutes

INGREDIENTS :

1 chicken breast cut into 2 x2 inch chunks

1 egg, whisked

1/4 cup almond flour

2 tbsps. onion powder

2 tbsps. garlic powder

1 tsp. dried oregano

1 tsp. paprika powder

1 tsp. salt

1/2 tsp. black pepper

2 tbsps. avocado oil

DIRECTIONS :

1. In a big bowl, combine all the dried ingredients. Mix well.

2. Place the eggs into a separate bowl.

3. Dip each chicken piece into the egg and then into the dry ingredients.

4. Heat oil in a 10-inch skillet, add oil.

5. Once avocado oil is hot, place the coated chicken nuggets onto a skillet and cook for 6-8 minutes until cooked and golden brown.

6. Serve with waffles and raspberries.

7. Enjoy!

NUTRITION :

Calories 401Kcal Fats 219g Protein 32.35g Net Carbs 1.46g

Crunchy Fish And Chaffle Bites

Servings :4

Cooking Time : 15 Minutes

INGREDIENTS :

1 lb. cod fillets, sliced into 4 slice

1 tsp. sea salt

1 tsp. garlic powder

1 egg, whisked

1 cup almond flour

2 tbsp. avocado oil

CHAFFLE INGREDIENTS :

2 eggs

1/2 cup cheddar cheese

2 tbsps. almond flour

½ tsp. Italian seasoning

DIRECTIONS :

1. Mix together chaffle ingredients in a bowl and make 4 square

2. Put the chaffles in a preheated chaffle maker.

3. Mix together the salt, pepper, and garlic powder in a mixing bowl. Toss the cod cubes in this mixture and let sit for 10 minutes.

4. Then dip each cod slice into the egg mixture and then into the almond flour.

5. Heat oil in skillet and fish cubes for about 2-3 minutes, until cooked and browned

6. Serve on chaffles and enjoy!

NUTRITION :

Protein: 121Kcal Fat: 189Kcal Carbohydrates: 11kcal

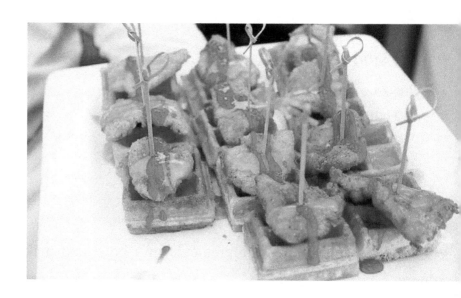

Grill Pork Waffle Sandwich

Servings :2

Cooking Time : 15 Minutes

INGREDIENTS :

1/2 cup mozzarella, shredded

1 egg

I pinch garlic powder

PORK PATTY

1/2 cup pork, minutesced

1 tbsp. green onion, diced

1/2 tsp Italian seasoning

Lettuce leaves

DIRECTIONS :

1. Preheat the square waffle maker and grease with

2. Mix together egg, cheese and garlic powder in a small mixing bowl.

3. Pour batter in a preheated waffle maker and cover.

4. Make 2 waffles from this batter.

5. Cook chaffles for about 2-3 minutes until cooked through.

6. Meanwhile, mix together pork patty ingredients in a bowl and make 1 large patty.

7. Grill pork patty in a preheated grill for about 3-4 minutes per side until cooked through.

8. Arrange pork patty between two chaffles with lettuce leaves. Cut the sandwich to make a triangular sandwich.

9. Enjoy!

NUTRITION :

Protein: 85Kcal Fat: 86Kcal Carbohydrates: 7Kcal

Chaffle & Chicken Lunch Plate

Servings :1

Cooking Time : 15 Minutes

INGREDIENTS :

1 large egg

1/2 cup jack cheese, shredded

1 pinch salt

For Serving

1 chicken leg

salt

pepper

1 tsp. garlic, minutesced

1 egg

I tsp avocado oil

DIRECTIONS :

1. Heat your square waffle maker and grease with cooking spray.

2. Pour Chaffle batter into the skillet and cook for about 3 minutes.

3. In a pan positioned on medium heat, heat the oil

4. Add chicken thigh and garlic in the oil then, cook for about 5 minutes. Flip and cook for another 3-4 minutes.

5. Season with salt and pepper and give them a good mix.

6. Transfer cooked thigh to plate.

7. Fry the egg in the same pan for about 1-2 minutes.

8. Once chaffles are cooked, serve with fried egg and chicken thigh

9. Enjoy!

NUTRITION :

Protein: 31% Fat: 66% Carbohydrates: 2%

Keto Lemon Chaffle Recipe

Preparation time: 5 minutes

Cooking time: 5 minutes

Servings : 4

INGREDIENTS :

Chaffle Cake:

2 tsp butter melted

1 tsp monk fruit powdered blend (add more if you like it sweeter)

1 tsp baking powder

2 eggs

2 tbsp coconut flour 2 oz cream cheese room temp and softened

1/2 tsp lemon extract

20 drops cake batter extract

Chaffle Frosting:

1/2 cup heavy whipping cream

1 tbsp monk fruit powdered confectioners blend 1/4 tsp lemon extract

DIRECTIONS :

Preheat the mini waffles machine

Apply all the chaffle cake ingredients to a blender and mix until the batter is smooth.

Using an ice cream scoop and using one full scoop of batter to fill the waffle iron.

Start making the frosting when the chaffles are boiling.

Apply the chaffle frosting ingredients to a medium-size dish.

Combine the components until the frosting is dense with peaks.

All the chaffles have to cool completely until the cake is frosted. Optional: For extra taste, add lemon peel!

NUTRITION :

Total Fat 20.3g Cholesterol 146.1mg Total Carbohydrate 5.2g Protein 5.6g

Bacon Cheddar Bay Biscuits Chaffle Recipe

Preparation time: 5 minutes
Cooking time: 7 minutes
Servings : 6

INGREDIENTS :

1/2 cup Almond Flour

1/4 cup Oat Fiber

1 1/2 T Kerrygold Butter melted

1/2 cup Sharp Cheddar Cheese shredded

3 strips of bacon cooked and crumbled

1/4 tsp Swerve Confectioners

1/2 tsp Garlic Salt

1/2 tsp Onion Powder

1/2 T Parsley dried

1T Bacon Grease melted

1/2 T Baking Powder

1 Egg, beat

1/2 cup Smoked Gouda Cheese shredded

1/4 tsp Baking Soda

1/4 cup Sour Cream

DIRECTIONS :

Prepare the Mini waffle maker for preheating

In a cup, whisk together the almond flour, baking powder, baking soda, onion powder, and garlic salt and combine

Add the eggs, bacon, sour cream, parsley, bacon grease, melted butter and cheese to another dish. Until paired, blend.

Connect the dry ingredients to the wet mixture and blend.

Spoon 2-3 tablespoons of the mixture into a warm waffle iron and cook for 5-6 minutes.

NUTRITION :

Total Fat 12.5g Total Carbohydrate 4.3g Protein 7.7g

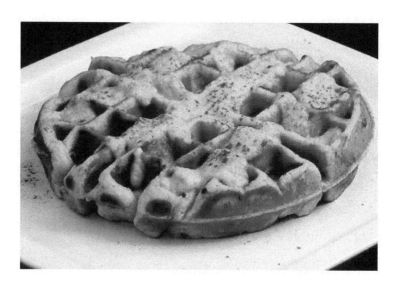

Lime Pie Chaffle Recipe

Preparation time: 5 minutes

Cooking time: 10 minutes

Servings : 2

INGREDIENTS :

1 egg

1/4 cup Almond flour

2 tsp cream cheese room temp

4 tbsp butter

1 tsp powdered sweetener swerve or monk fruit

1/2 tsp lime zest

1/2 tsp baking powder

Pinch of salt

1/2 tsp lime zest

Cream Cheese Lime Frosting ingredients:

4 oz cream cheese softened

2 tsp powdered sweetener swerve or monk fruit

1 tsp lime extract

1/2 tsp lime extract

DIRECTIONS :

Preheat the iron with the mini waffle.

Add all the chaffle components to a blender and blend until smooth.

Cook each chaffle until golden brown for approximately 3 to 4 minutes. Make the frosting when the chaffles are boiling.

Mix all the frosting ingredients in a small bowl and mix until it is smooth. Before frosting them, cause the chaffles to fully cool.

NUTRITION :

Total Fat 5.7g Total Carbohydrate 4.9g Protein 5.5g

Jicama Hash Brown Chaffle

Preparation time: 5 minutes

Cooking time: 10 minutes

Servings : 4

INGREDIENTS :

1 large jicama root

1/2 medium onion minced

2 garlic cloves pressed

1 cup cheese of choice

2 eggs whisked

Salt and Pepper

DIRECTIONS :

Peel the jicama

Shred in processor for food

Sprinkle with 1-2 tsp of salt and put the shredded jicama in a large colander. Mix thoroughly and allow to drain.

Squeeze as much liquid as possible out of it. For 5-8 minutes, microwave.

Combine all ingredients

Before applying 3T of the mixture, sprinkle a little cheese on the waffle iron, and sprinkle a little more cheese on top of the mixture.

NUTRITION :

Total Fat 11.8g Total Carbohydrate 5.1g Protein 10g

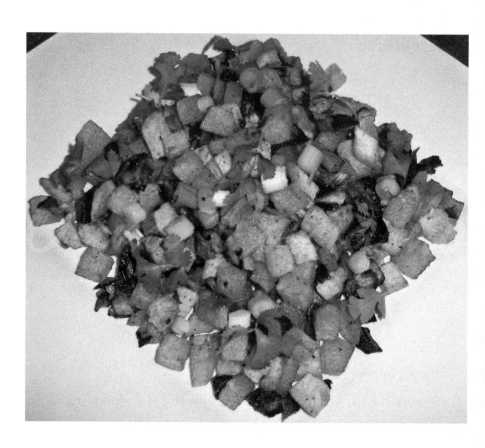

Easy Corndog Chaffle Recipe

Preparation time: 5 minutes

Cooking time: 10 minutes

Servings : 5

INGREDIENTS :

2 eggs

1 cup Mexican cheese blend

1 tbsp almond flour

1/2 tsp cornbread extract

1/4 tsp salt

hot dogs with hot dog sticks

DIRECTIONS :

Preheat the Waffle Maker for Corndog.

Whip the eggs in a small cup.

Except the hotdogs, add the remaining ingredients

Spray with non-stick cooking spray on the corn dog waffle maker. Fill the maker of corn dog waffles with the halfway filled batter. In the hot dog, put a stick.

Drop the hot dog in the batter and press down gently.

Spread a little more on top of the hot dog, just enough to fill it up. Makes about 4 to 5 corndogs for chaffle.

For 4 minutes, cook the corn dog waffles.

When finished, they are quickly removed with a pair of tongs from the corn dog waffle maker. Serve with mustard, mayo, or ketchup that is sugar-free!

NUTRITION :

Total Fat 5.5g Total Carbohydrate 1.8g Protein 6.8g

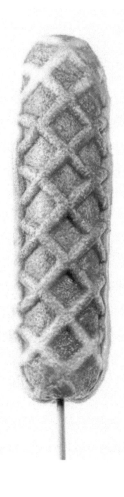

Sloppy Joe Chaffle Recipe

Preparation time: 5 minutes

Cooking time: 10 minutes

INGREDIENTS :

Sloppy Joe ingredients:

1 lb ground beef

1 tsp garlic minced

3 tbsp tomato paste

1 tbsp chili powder

1 tsp cocoa powder optional

1/2 cup bone broth beef flavor

1/2 tsp salt

1 tsp onion powder

1/4 tsp pepper

1 tsp Swerve brown

1/2 tsp paprika

1 tsp mustard powder

1 tsp coconut aminos or soy sauce

Cornbread Chaffle ingredients:

Makes 2 chaffles

1/4 tsp corn extract optional but tastes like real cornbread!

1/2 cup cheddar cheese

1 egg

5 slices jalapeno diced very small (can be pickled or fresh)

1 tsp Franks Red Hot Sauce

Pinch salt

DIRECTIONS :

First of all, cook the ground beef with salt and pepper. All the remaining ingredients are added

Enable the mixture to boil while the chaffles are being made. Waffle maker for preheating

Whip the egg in a tiny tub.

The remaining ingredients are added.

Using nonstick cooking oil, spray the waffle maker. Break the mixture in half.

Cook half the mixture for 4 minutes or until golden brown.

Before applying the mixture, add 1 tsp of cheese to the waffle maker for 30 seconds for a crunchy outer crust on the chaffle.

Onto a hot chaffle, pour the warm sloppy joe mix.

Keto Smores Chaffle

Servings : 2

INGREDIENTS :

Pinch of pink salt

2 tbsp swerve brown

2 tbsp Keto Marshmallow Creme Fluff Recipe

1 large Egg

½ tbs Psyllium Husk Powder optional

¼ tsp Baking Powder

½ c. Mozzarella cheese shredded

½ tsp Vanilla extract

¼ Lily's Original Dark Chocolate Bar

DIRECTIONS :

Create a Keto Marshmallow Creme Fluff batch. Whisk until creamy with the egg.

Combine vanilla with Swerve Brown and blend well.

Mix and blend in the shredded cheese.

Then add the baking powder, Psyllium Husk Powder, and salt. Mix until well incorporated, 3-4 minutes to let the batter rest. Prep/plug in to preheat your waffle maker.

Spread the waffle maker with ½ batter and cook for 3-4 minutes. Remove and set on a rack for cooling.

Cook the same batter for the second half, then remove to cool.

Assemble the chaffles with the marshmallow fluff and chocolate until they are cool: use 2 tbs of marshmallow and ¼ bar of Lily's Chocolate.

For a melty and gooey S'more sandwich, eat as is, or toast!

NUTRITION (per serving):

Total Fat 8.1g Total Carbohydrate 3.1g Protein 8.3g

Pumpkin Chaffle With Cream Cheese Frosting

Servings : 3

INGREDIENTS :

1 egg

1 tbsp pumpkin solid packed with no sugar added

1/2 cup mozzarella cheese

1/2 tsp pumpkin pie spice

Optional Cream Cheese Frosting ingredients:

2 tbsp monk fruit confectioners blend or any of your favorite keto-friendly sweetener 1/2 tsp clear vanilla extract

2 tbsp cream cheese softened and room temperature

DIRECTIONS :

Preheat the mini waffle machine.

Whip the egg in a tiny tub.

Connect the cheese, spice for the pumpkin pie, and the pumpkin.

Mix thoroughly.

In the mini waffle maker, add 1/2 of the mixture and cook it for at least 3 to 4 minutes until it is golden brown.

Add all the cream cheese frosting ingredients to a bowl while the chaffle is cooking and mix until it's smooth and fluffy.

Attach a frosting of cream cheese to the hot chaffle and serve immediately.

NUTRITION :

Calories 84 Total Fat 4.5g Total Carbohydrate 5.3g Protein 6.1g

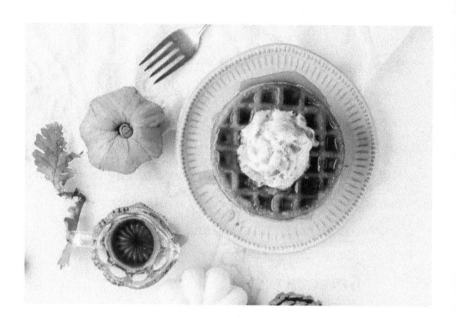

Lightning Source UK Ltd.
Milton Keynes UK
UKHW020745250621
386136UK00005B/88

9 781803 178516